ILEOSTOMY DIET COOKBOOK

Designing an Ileostomy Diet that Fits Your Lifestyle

Balancing Nutrition And Flavor For Long-Term Well-Being

Dr. Elias Elizabeth

CHAPTER ONE

Introduction

Living with an ileostomy may be a life-changing event, forcing people to adjust to a new way of life. An ileostomy is a surgical treatment that involves diverting a portion of the small intestine through a hole in the abdominal wall, resulting in a stoma.

This stoma acts as a waste exit, hence an ostomy pouch is required to collect bodily waste. While physical and mental changes may be difficult, knowing and managing food concerns is an important element of post-ileostomy life.

A personalized diet becomes essential for ileostomy patients to ensure they get appropriate nutrition while negotiating any food limitations. In this examination, we will look at the complexities of ileostomy, the advantages of a personalized diet, and how people may satisfy their nutritional demands while dealing with this transformational surgical operation.

Understanding Ileostomy

An ileostomy is commonly accomplished when a section of the small intestine, known as the ileum, is brought to the surface of the abdomen to produce a stoma. This surgical operation is often required in response to a variety of medical disorders, including inflammatory bowel disease, colon cancer, or digestive system injuries.

The stoma serves as a fresh exit point for waste, enabling it to skip the lower digestive tract. Ileostomy surgery may be temporary or permanent, depending on the underlying medical condition and the patient's requirements.

Individuals who have had ileostomy surgery experience major changes in their everyday life. Aside from the bodily changes, there are emotional and psychological implications to consider. Patients may feel unsure, self-conscious, or anxious about managing their bodily functions with an ostomy pouch. Understanding the importance of a personalized diet in supporting general health and well-being is an important step toward smoothing this transition.

Benefits of Tailored Diets

Individuals with an ileostomy should follow a specialized diet that addresses their unique nutritional demands and promotes digestive health. One of the most significant advantages of following a personalized diet is the ability to reduce problems associated with an ileostomy, such as dehydration, electrolyte imbalance, and malnutrition. Ileostomy patients may improve their overall quality of life by being mindful of their food choices.

The focus on readily digested meals is an important part of an ileostomy-specific diet. Because the digestive system experiences major changes after surgery, it is important to consume meals that are soft on the digestive tract.

This often entails integrating well-cooked and softer foods into the diet, such as steamed vegetables, lean meats, and easily digested cereals. Staying hydrated is also important since people with ileostomies are more likely to lose fluid via the stoma.

Navigating Dietary Restrictions

While a personalized diet is vital for ileostomy patients, overcoming possible dietary limitations is just as critical. Certain meals might cause problems for people with an ileostomy, such as blockages, gas, or diarrhea. High-fiber diets, for example, maybe more difficult to digest, resulting in greater stool production. Foods known to induce gas, such as beans and cruciferous vegetables, should also be ingested in moderation.

Ileostomy patients must collaborate with healthcare specialists, especially nutritionists and ostomy nurses, to discover specific food triggers and limits. Keeping a food diary may be a useful tool in this process, allowing people to monitor their dietary choices and find trends associated with ostomy function. Patients who recognize and avoid hazardous meals might reduce their risk of problems and live a more pleasant and predictable lifestyle.

CHAPTER TWO

Essential Nutrients for Ileostomy Patients

Maintaining an appropriate diet is critical for people with ileostomies since the surgical procedure might affect nutrient absorption and utilization. Key nutrients, such as vitamins and minerals, are essential for general health and recovery. Ileostomy patients should pay close attention to the following critical nutrients:

1. Electrolytes: Ileostomy patients may have increased fluid and electrolyte loss via the stoma. Maintaining fluid balance, sustaining nerve function, and avoiding dehydration all need adequate electrolyte intake.

2. Protein is required for tissue regeneration and maintenance, making it an important part of the post-ileostomy

diet. Lean protein sources, such as chicken, fish, eggs, and tofu, may aid in the healing process and prevent muscle wastage.

3. Vitamins and minerals: Some vitamins and minerals, including as vitamin B12, iron, and calcium, may be less well absorbed by ileostomy patients. Regular nutritional monitoring and, if required, supplementation may help avoid deficiencies and promote general health.

4. Fluids: Staying hydrated is critical for those with ileostomies. Increased fluid intake may help prevent dehydration induced by the stoma's elevated fluid outflow. Water, herbal teas, and electrolyte-rich drinks are great options for staying hydrated.

Finally, adjusting to life with an ileostomy requires more than just physical changes; it also takes a careful approach to nutritional choices. A personalized diet for ileostomy patients has various advantages, ranging from reducing problems to improving general health and well-being. Navigating dietary limitations becomes critical in this journey, as people learn to recognize and manage items that may cause problems after surgery.

Ileostomy patients may improve their nutritional intake, help the healing process, and live a happy life outside of the limits of their surgical intervention by emphasizing important nutrients. Individuals with an ileostomy may achieve resilience, adaptation, and long-term well-being by receiving information, collaborating with healthcare providers, and committing to a well-balanced diet.

Living with an ileostomy may provide unique obstacles, particularly in terms of maintaining a healthy and pleasurable diet. However, with careful preparation and imagination, you may tailor your ileostomy meal plan to be both tasty and nutrient-dense. This entails modifying recipes, planning meals, and including snacks that are not only tasty but also easy on your digestion.

Customizing Your Ileostomy Diet Plan

Customizing your ileostomy food plan is essential for maintaining your overall health. The first step is to understand your dietary requirements and any limits indicated by your healthcare provider. Every person's body reacts differently to various foods, so it's important to pay attention to how you feel after each meal.

Consider speaking with a qualified dietician who specializes in assisting people with ostomies. They may provide tailored guidance and assist you in developing a food plan that fits your nutritional needs while taking into consideration any restrictions imposed by your ileostomy.

When designing your diet, include a range of nutrient-dense foods such as fruits, vegetables, lean meats, and whole grains. These foods may give necessary vitamins and minerals, hence improving general health. Furthermore, keeping hydrated is critical for ileostomy patients, who may be more susceptible to dehydration owing to increased fluid loss.

Creating Flavorful and Nutritious Meals

One widespread myth concerning ileostomy diets is that they must be bland and limiting. However, there are several methods to prepare delectable and nutrient-dense meals while meeting your unique dietary requirements.

Experiment with herbs and spices to improve the flavor of your food without using excessive salt or fat. Fresh herbs like basil, cilantro, and mint, as well as spices like turmeric, cumin, and paprika, may enhance the depth and taste of your dishes.

Include a variety of colored fruits and vegetables in your diet to acquire a wide range of nutrients. These may be cooked or eaten raw, according to your tastes and tolerances. Steaming, roasting, or sautéing vegetables may improve their flavor and digestibility.

Choose lean foods like chicken, turkey, fish, and tofu to provide your protein needs without creating digestive distress. Grilling or baking these proteins may be a tasty and healthier alternative to frying.

Incorporate healthy grains such as quinoa, brown rice, and oats into your meals to increase your fiber intake. Fiber is vital for digestive health, and many people with ileostomies handle whole grains well.

CHAPTER THREE

Adapting recipes for ileostomy-friendly cooking

Adapting recipes for ileostomy-friendly cooking entails making mindful replacements and adaptations to meet your specific dietary requirements. Consider utilizing low-fiber substitutes for certain products to reduce the risk of clogs or discomfort.

If high-fiber meals aggravate your digestive troubles, choose refined grains over whole grains. Similarly, choose well-cooked and peeled fruits and vegetables to lower fiber content while keeping nutritional value.

Experiment with different flavors, such as substituting low-residue sauces or broths for heavy or spicy seasonings. Be wary of foods that are known to induce gas, since too much gas may be painful for ileostomy patients.

It's also critical to watch meal amounts to prevent overwhelming your digestive system. Eating smaller, more frequent meals throughout the day may help you stay energized without overloading your digestive system.

Meal Planning and Preparation Tips

Successful ileostomy diet plans need effective meal planning and preparation. To simplify the procedure and guarantee a balanced nutritional intake, consider the following suggestions:

1. Plan: Set aside some time each week to plan your meals and snacks. This allows you to make more educated judgments and prevent last-minute decisions that may result in less-than-ideal dietary alternatives.

2. Prepare your fruits, veggies, and proteins ahead of time by washing, chopping, and portioning them. Having prepared foods on hand may make meals more efficient and stress-free.

3. Batch cooking involves preparing bigger amounts of meals and freezing them in individual pieces. This is particularly useful on days when you may not have the energy or time to prepare.

4. Use Convenience Meals Wisely: While fresh, whole meals are best, there's nothing wrong with adopting certain convenience goods, such as pre-cut veggies or pre-cooked grains, to save time and effort.

5. Stay Hydrated: Drink lots of fluids throughout the day. Dehydration is a problem for ileostomy patients, so make an effort to stay hydrated.

Snack Ideas for Ileostomy Patients

Snacking may be an important element of an ileostomy diet, giving extra nutrients and energy in between meals. However, it's important to choose foods that are easy for your digestive system. Here are some snack options designed for ileostomy sufferers.

1. Yogurt with Soft Fruit: Combine low-fat, plain yogurt with soft fruits such as bananas or strawberries. This offers a balance of protein and natural sweetness.

2. Nut Butter and Crackers: Spread almond or peanut butter on low-fiber crackers for a tasty and protein-packed snack.

3. Smoothies: Combine ripe bananas, yogurt, and a dash of fruit juice to make a delicious and easily digested smoothie.

4. Cheese and Grapes: For a well-balanced protein and natural sugar intake, pair modest quantities of cheese with seedless grapes.

5. Hard-boiled eggs are a simple and protein-rich snack. Season with a touch of salt and pepper for more taste.

6. Hummus with Carrot Sticks: Serve hummus with peeled and sliced carrot sticks for a delicious and healthy snack.

7. Rice Cakes with Avocado: Top rice cakes with mashed avocado for a simple and filling snack that is easy on the stomach.

You can enjoy a diverse and satisfying diet while supporting your overall health and well-being by customizing your ileostomy diet plan, creating flavorful and nutrient-rich meals, adapting recipes for ileostomy-friendly cooking, carefully planning and preparing meals, and incorporating gentle snacks.

CHAPTER FOUR

Drink Options for Optimal Hydration

Hydration is a critical component in maintaining overall health and wellness. The beverages we consume daily have a significant impact on our hydration levels. Water is, of course, the most important source of hydration, but other drinks may also add to our fluid intake. The goal is to make deliberate decisions that meet our bodies' water requirements.

Water remains the foundation of hydration. It is calorie-free, easily accessible, and required for a variety of biological activities. Drinking enough of water helps regulate body temperature, carry nutrients, and wash away waste materials. Aim to drink at least eight 8-ounce glasses of water every day, although individual requirements may vary depending on age, activity level, and environment.

In addition to water, herbal teas may be both hydrating and tasty. Herbal teas, like peppermint or chamomile, not only give diversity to your beverage options, but they also have possible health advantages. Caffeinated drinks, such as coffee and black tea, may have a diuretic effect, possibly causing greater fluid loss.

Sports drinks are intended to replace electrolytes lost during strenuous physical exercise. While they may be useful for athletes who participate in lengthy, strenuous activities, they may not be required for the normal individual.

To remain hydrated without the additional sweets found in commercial sports drinks, drink water or make your electrolyte drink by blending water, a bit of salt, and a splash of citrus juice.

Eating out with confidence

Dining out is a typical occurrence in contemporary life, and choosing healthy choices when dining out may be difficult. However, with enough organization and attention, you can confidently navigate restaurant menus.

Begin by examining the menu for healthier selections. Look for meals with lean meats, nutritious grains, and a range of colorful veggies. Many restaurants now include nutritional information for their menu items, allowing you to make educated decisions regarding calorie and nutrient intake.

When placing an order, consider the portion sizes. Restaurants often provide greater amounts than required for a single meal. Choose lesser amounts or split a meal with a dining buddy. Alternatively, ask for a to-go box at the start of the meal and put away a part of your food before you begin eating to prevent overindulging.

Be wary of cooking procedures. Grilled, baked, or steamed foods are often healthier than fried or highly sautéed ones. To keep your consumption under control, ask for dressings and sauces on the side.

Managing Special Occasions and Social Events

Special celebrations and social activities often focus on food, making it difficult to maintain good eating habits. However, with a deliberate approach, you may enjoy these times without jeopardizing your well-being.

Before attending an event, eat a modest, balanced meal or snack to satisfy hunger and avoid overindulgence. Choose nutrient-dense meals that give long-term energy, such as protein, fiber, and healthy fats.

Practice mindful eating during social gatherings. Pay attention to hunger and fullness signs, and enjoy every mouthful. Choose meals that you appreciate rather than simply trying everything offered.

Moderation is crucial. Allow yourself to enjoy exceptional delicacies, but be cautious of portion proportions. Consider sharing desserts or ordering a smaller piece to fulfill your appetites without overindulging.

CHAPTER FIVE

Fitness and Nutrition for Long-Term Wellness

The integration of activity and nutrition is critical for reaching and sustaining long-term well-being. Regular physical exercise and a well-balanced diet help to improve general health and avoid chronic illnesses.

To improve total fitness, do a variety of aerobic, strength, and flexibility activities. Find things that you like to make fitness a regular part of your routine. Staying active, whether by walking, cycling, swimming, or dancing, helps with weight control, mood improvement, and cardiovascular health.

Nutrition is the fuel that drives your body through physical exercise and everyday living. Prioritize a well-balanced diet that includes fruits, vegetables, whole grains, lean meats, and healthy fats. Balance is essential, and portion control is critical for weight management.

Consider working with a qualified nutritionist or fitness expert to develop a tailored strategy that meets your health objectives. They may advise you on calorie requirements, nutritional consumption, and activities geared to your personal needs and tastes.

Mindful Eating and Emotional Wellness

Mindful eating entails paying attention to the sensory aspects of food, such as taste, texture, and smell. It also entails being mindful of hunger and fullness signals and selecting foods that support both physical and emotional well-being.

Emotional well-being has a huge impact on our relationship with food. Stress, boredom, and other emotions may all impact eating patterns, leading to overeating or making poor choices. Developing skills to deal with emotions without resorting to food is critical for long-term well-being.

Slowing down throughout meals promotes attentive eating. Chew your meal deeply, relish each mouthful, and avoid distractions such as television or technological gadgets when eating. This might help you become more aware of your body's cues of hunger and fullness.

If emotional eating is a problem, explore other strategies to deal with stress or unpleasant emotions. This might involve deep breathing exercises, meditation, or indulging in hobbies that offer you pleasure and contentment.

Conclusion

Incorporating these principles into your everyday routine will help you take a more holistic approach to your health and well-being. Making mindful beverage choices, confidently dining out, managing special events, prioritizing exercise and nutrition, and cultivating mindful eating behaviors all contribute to your long-term health objectives.

By adopting a proactive and balanced approach to these parts of your life, you may develop habits that will lead to a healthier, happier, and more satisfying existence.